VITAL PREGNANCY CHECKLIST

A Complete Pictorial Guide for Nursing Mothers and Pregnant Women in Preparation For Newborns

By

Helen Romero

Table of Contents

CHAPTER ONE

What's the essence of this book?

Let me give you a short story of my pregnancy moment, being a young lady getting married to the love of my life was the best thing that ever happened to me, butterflies all caught up in my stomach, I pleasured them like it was never going to end. Quite soon we got a new addition it wasn't a child's play. Indeed I clamored how my mom was able to handle me and my siblings. Few months to the day of my delivery, we embarked on shopping for our unborn baby, we got some details from my mom on what to get.

More confusion set in as we started the purchase, more than one hour we went back and forth on whether we bought the right things or if the quantity was enough. That day was never to forget, guess what we stayed longer than four hours, checking the internet and the list to see if they matched. Thanks to a kind-hearted saleswoman who assisted us in getting it done, she had two kids already, so her experience level was welcoming. Back home I sat and thought of how other women would go through this stress to get their nursing list checked.

With a thoughtful heart, I went through the rigors to put this book in line with minimal words and more of images depicting the items needed. I hope you enjoy this piece, thank you. Let's move to class our intending couples, single parents, and married ones.

CHAPTER TWO

What should be in your checklist?

Basically the items and quantities written below serves as a guide, meaning it's flexible, therefore you have the freewill.

Feeding Tools

- Lots of bibs
- Burp cloths
- Breast pump
- Milk storage containers
- Nursing pillow
- Nursing bras (not yet given birth get one that is adjustable)
- Breast pads (disposable or washable)
- Lotion for sore nipples

Mother's Formula Feeding Tools

- Lots of bibs
- Burp cloths
- Six 120ml Baby bottles with nipples
- Six 60ml Baby bottles with nipples
- Bottle and nipple brush

- Baby formula, check for ingredients, batch number and expiry date
- Thermal bottle carrier

Diapering Tools: Re-usable Diaper Hints
- Up to 10 cloth or re-usable diapers
- Five waterproof covers
- One or two Baby Diaper Genie
- Two or three Changing pad
- Smooth baby ointment to prevent rash
- Safety pins to fasten re-usable diapers
- Six disposable wipes or six washcloths for cleaning baby's buttocks

Disposable diapers in use
- One box of newborn diapers, don't buy excess weight to prevent wastage because your baby's weight might change
- One Baby Diaper Genie
- Two or three Changing pad
- Smooth baby ointment to prevent rash
- Six disposable wipes or six washcloths for cleaning baby's bottom

Clothing

- Ten undershirts (blend of short and long sleeves)
- Six nightgowns (ensure the cord falls off before use)
- Eight one-piece stretchy sleepers (purchase with zippers)
- Five pairs of pants
- Three newborn hats
- Six pairs of socks to wear with nightgowns and outfits
- Two pairs of scratch mittens, to keep baby from scratching his face
- Three cardigans more in winter
- Bunting bag for winter baby
- Detergent for infants
- Three outfits for dressing up

Blankets

- Three large cotton blankets
- Six receiving blankets (they also make handy burp cloths)

Bath time

- One plastic infant tub

- Ten washcloths, not used on baby's buttocks
- Gentle baby soap
- One or two soft-bristled hair brush
- Two Soft-hooded towels

Bedtime: When using a crib

- Dedicated crib and crib mattress for baby
- Three waterproof mattress covers
- Three fitted crib sheets
- Three light blankets that fit in the crib
- Two Sleep sack

When mother sleeps side by side with baby

- Firm mattress (don't use waterbed)
- Three fitted crib sheets
- Three waterproof pads to place under baby
- One or more Light comforter
- Sleep sack

Additional items

- Dedicated infant safety seat for car
- Reclined stroller, so baby can lie flat
- Baby nail clippers
- Six Bulb syringe for mucous suctioning
- Baby thermometer
- Eye dropper
- Medicine spoon

More value to caring

- Change table or change pad
- Rocking chair that supports feeding and swaddling
- Good playpen
- Sling carrier
- Diaper bag
- One or change pads
- Plastic hangers for baby closet
- Sun shield for car windows
- One or two pacifiers
- Baby toys
- Baby mobiles
- Baby night light

CHAPTER THREE

On the go pictorial presentation

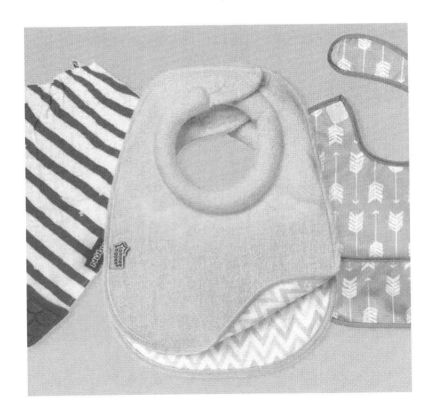

Baby bibs

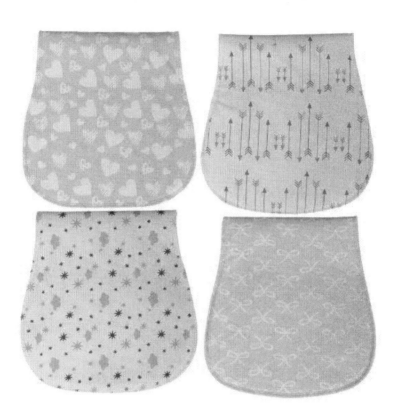

Burb clothes

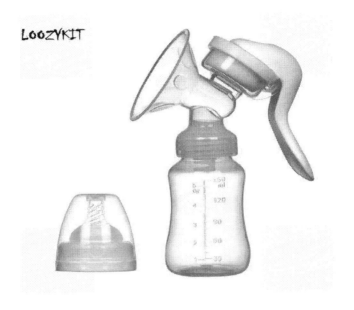

Breast pump

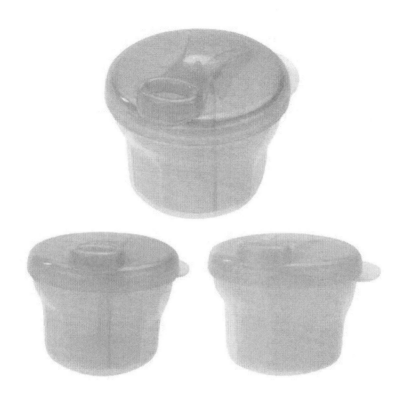

Milk storage containers

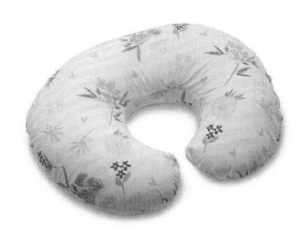

Nursing pillow

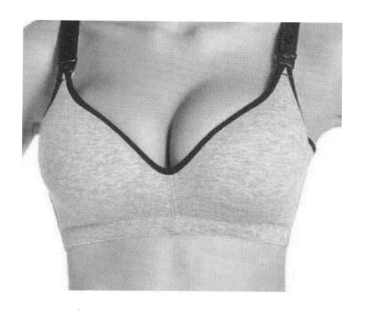

Nursing bras

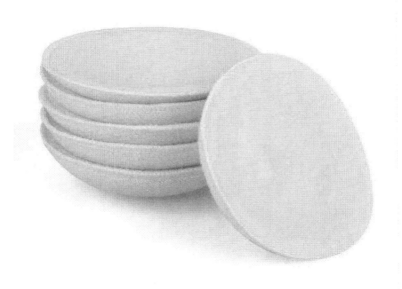

Breast pads

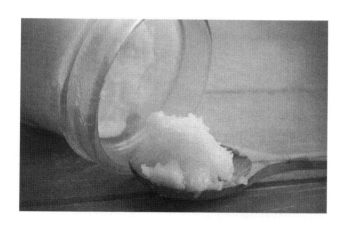

Lotion for sore nipples

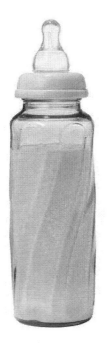

Baby bottles with nipples

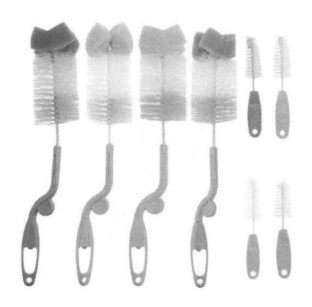

Bottle and nipple brush

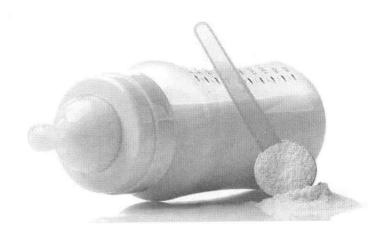

Baby formula

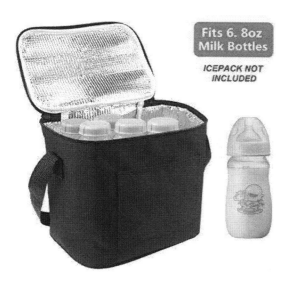

Fits 6. 8oz
Milk Bottles

*ICEPACK NOT
INCLUDED*

Thermal bottle carrier

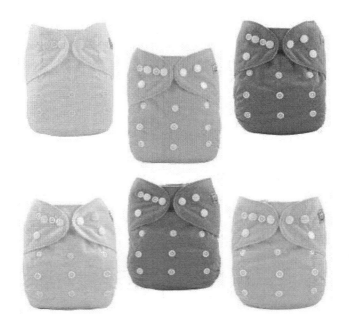

Re-usable diapers

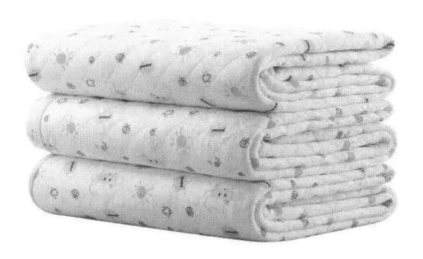

Waterproof covers

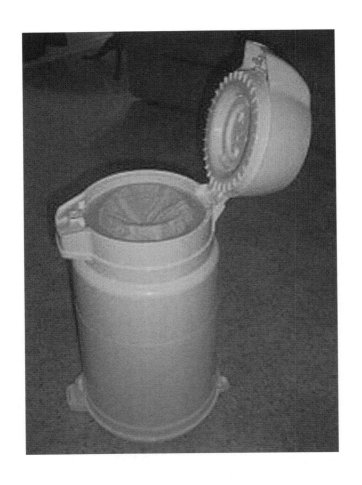

Baby Diaper Genie

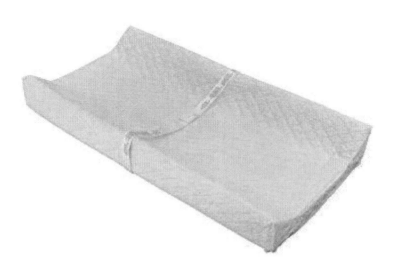

Changing pad

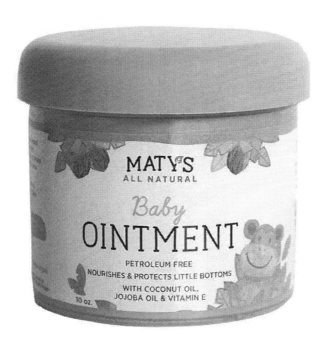

Baby ointment

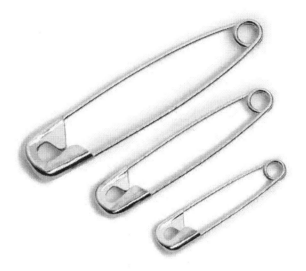

Safety pins

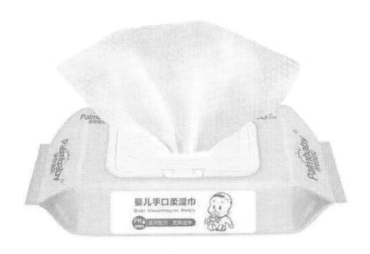

Disposable wipes

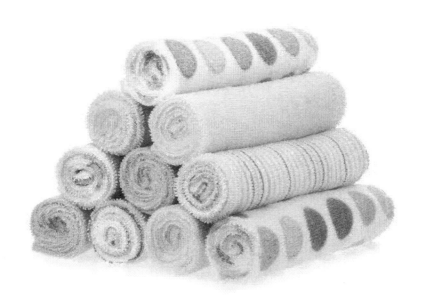

Wash clothes

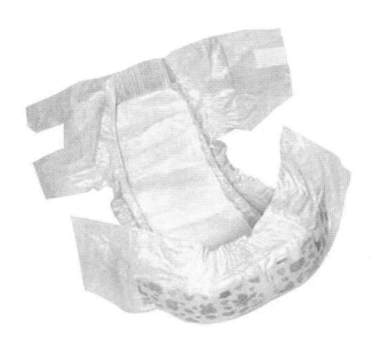

Disposable diapers

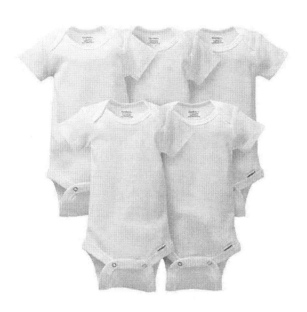

Undershirts

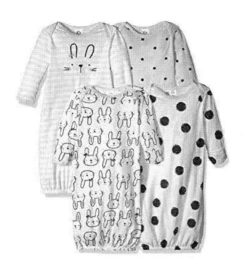

Nightgowns

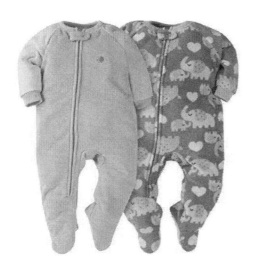

Stretchy sleepers

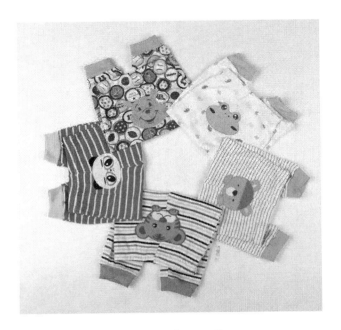

Pairs of pants

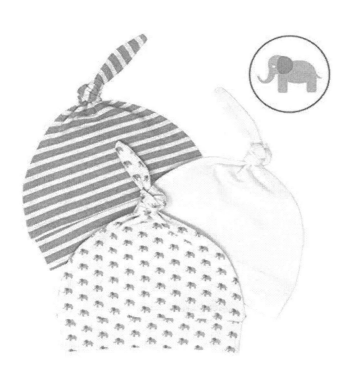

Newborn hats

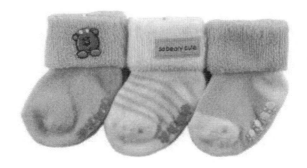

Pairs of socks

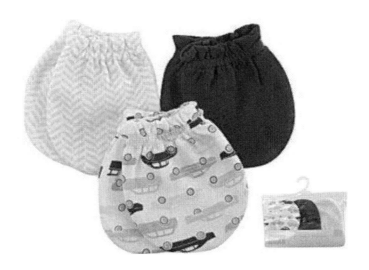

Scratch mittens

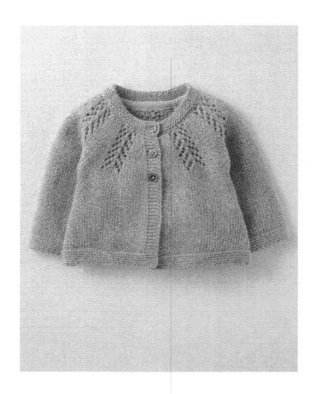

Cardigan

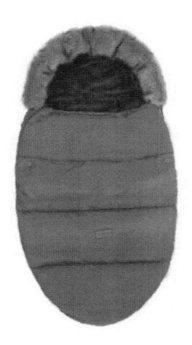

Bunting bag

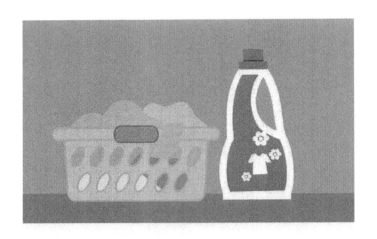

Detergent

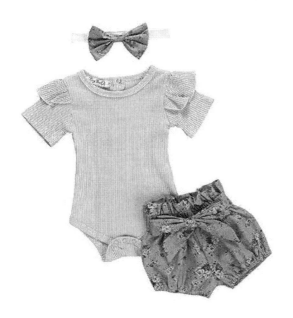

Outfits

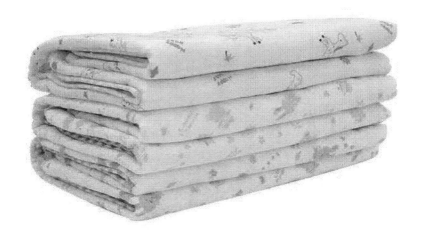

Cotton blankets

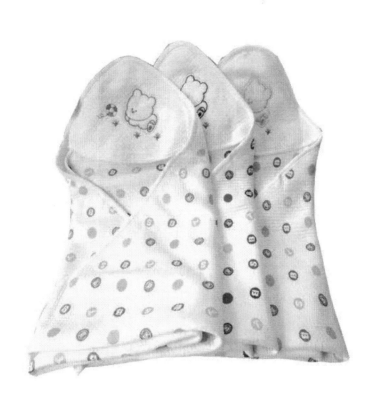

Receiving blankets

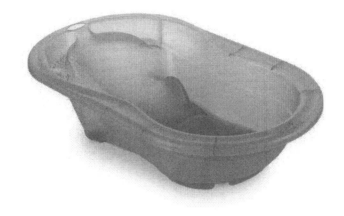

Plastic infant tub

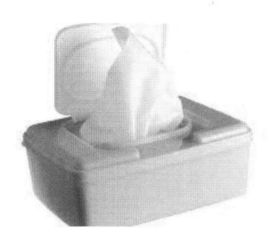

Washcloths (not used for buttocks)

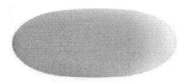

Baby soap

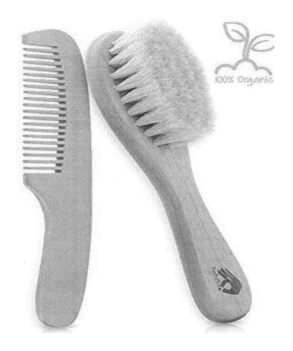

Soft-bristled hair brush

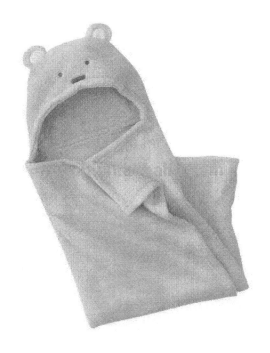

Soft-hooded towels

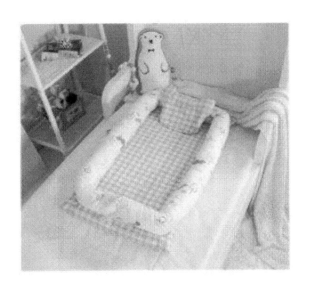

Crib and crib mattress

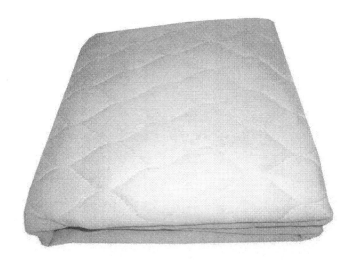

Waterproof mattress

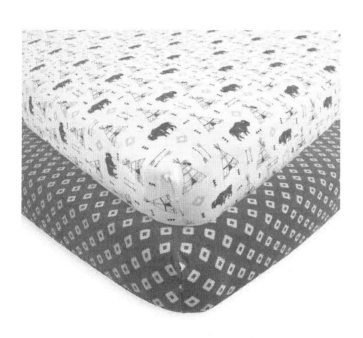

Fitted crib sheets

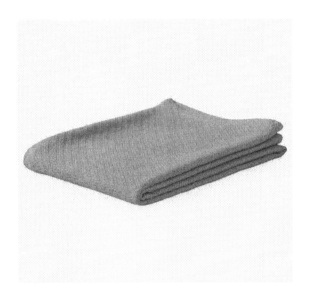

Light blankets

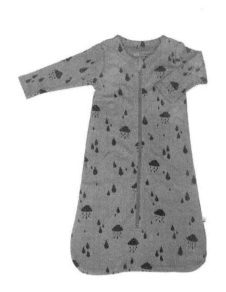

Sleep sack

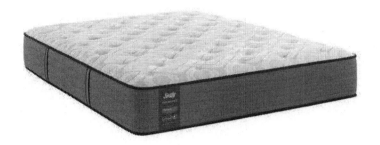

Firm mattress

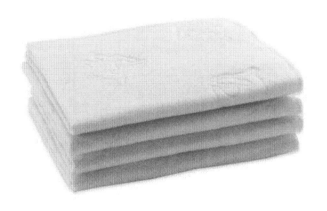

Waterproof pads

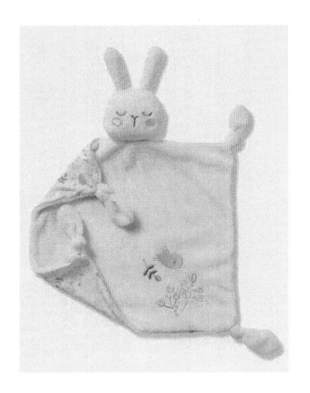

Light comforter

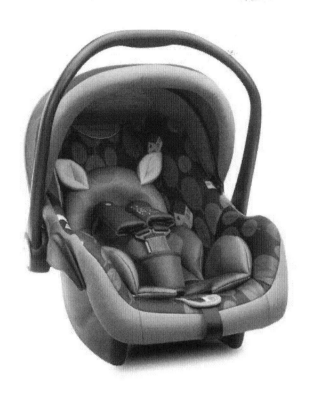

Infant safety seat

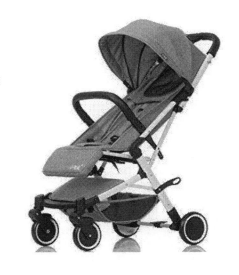

Reclined stroller

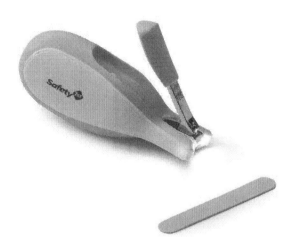

Nail clippers

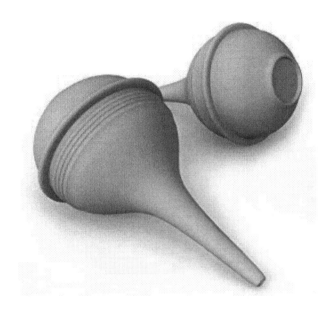

Bulb syringe

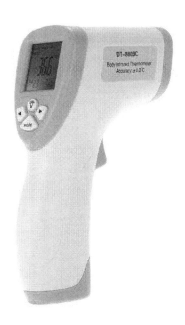

Baby thermometer

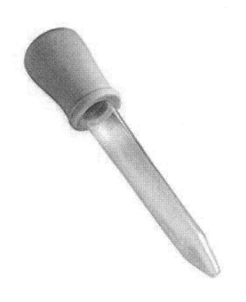

Eye dropper

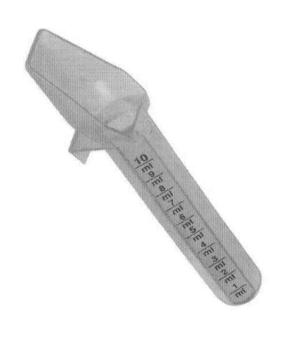

Medicine spoon

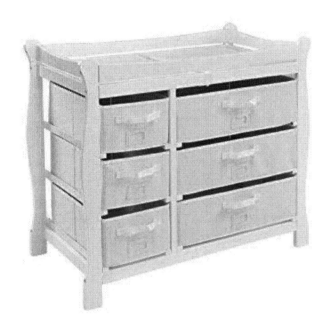

Change table

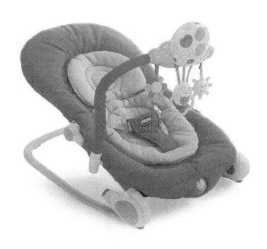

Rocking chair

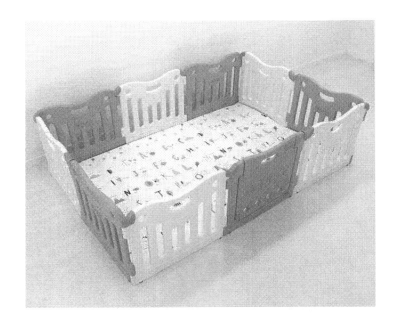

Good playpen

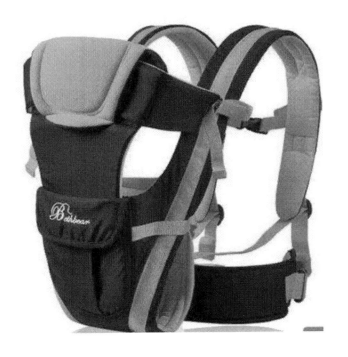

Sling carrier

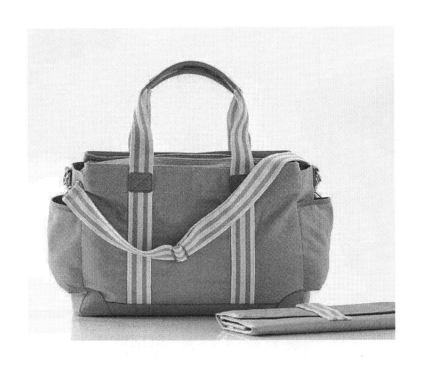

Diaper bag

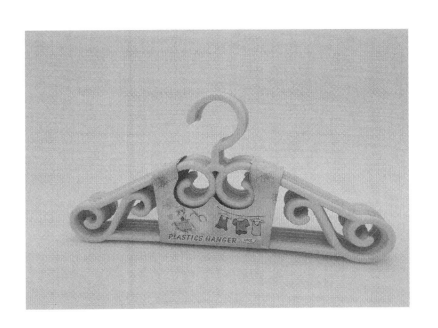

Plastic hangers

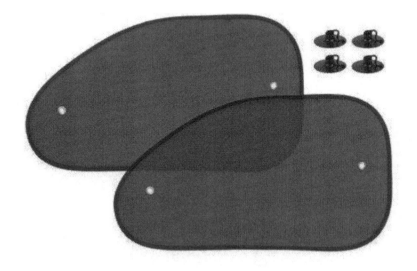

Sun shield

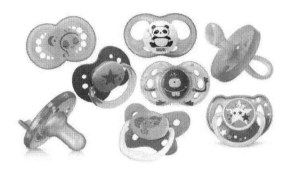

Pacifiers

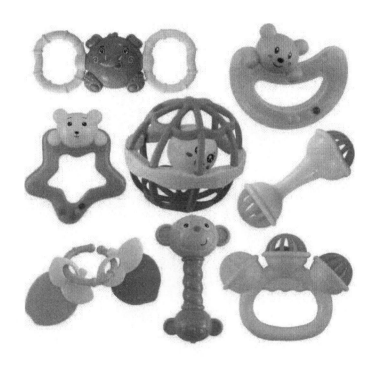

Baby toys

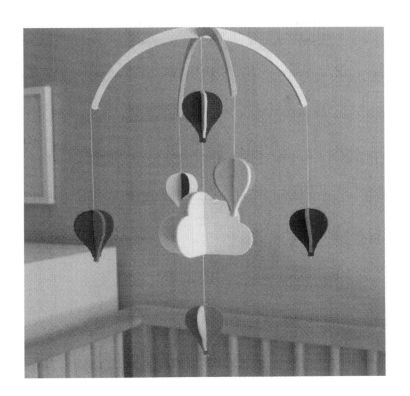

Baby mobiles

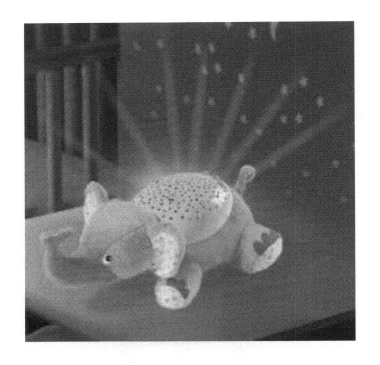

Night light

A BIG THANK YOU!!!

Printed in Great Britain
by Amazon

39004406R00045